Healing Hearts, Guiding Hands: Daily Devotionals For Physiotherapists

Delightful Devotionals

CONTENTS

Introduction

In the dynamic realm of physiotherapy, where the healing touch meets the intricacies of human anatomy, this devotional unfolds as a companion on your journey of compassionate care.

Over the next 21 days, we delve into the sacred fusion of spiritual reflection and the noble art of therapeutic practice.

Rooted in the foundational truths of scripture, this devotional serves as a source of inspiration and guidance for physiotherapists navigating the challenges and joys of their vital profession.

Physiotherapy is not just a vocation but a divine calling to participate in the restoration of health and well-being. This devotional invites you to embark on a reflective expedition, intertwining your daily practices with timeless biblical principles.

As you engage with each day's scripture, encouragement, and introspective questions, may you discover a deeper connection between your healing hands and the divine purpose that propels your work.

Through these pages, we explore the profound intersection of faith and the therapeutic journey, seeking to infuse your professional life with spiritual significance.

Amidst the demands of healthcare, this devotional aims to offer moments of solace, inspiration, and spiritual renewal. It serves as a reminder that your role as a physiotherapist extends beyond the physical, reaching into the realms of emotional and spiritual well-being.

Join this transformative journey, embracing the divine guidance that intertwines with the art and science of healing.

Day 1: The Gift of Healing Hands

Verse of the Day:

Isaiah 41:10 - "So do not fear, for I am with you; do not be dismayed, for I am your God. I will strengthen you and help you; I will uphold you with my righteous right hand."

Reflection:

In the realm of physiotherapy, your hands are more than instruments; they are conduits of healing grace. As you embark on your daily journey, remember the divine assurance in Isaiah 41:10.

Fear not, for God is with you, guiding your hands and infusing your work with strength. Your touch becomes an extension of the Almighty's comforting presence.

As you engage in the noble task of mending and restoring, take solace in the profound truth that God is your source of unwavering support. Your hands are upheld by the righteous right hand of the Creator.

Every gesture, every gentle touch, resonates with a divine promise of strength. Embrace the sacred nature of your calling, recognizing that through your hands, healing becomes a tangible expression of God's compassion.

Journal:

1. Reflect on a moment when you felt God's strength guiding your hands in your practice. How did it impact your work?

2. Consider instances where you have witnessed the profound effect of compassionate touch on your patients. How does it align with the scriptural promise in Isaiah 41:10?

3. In what ways can you intentionally incorporate prayer into your daily practice, seeking God's guidance and strength as you utilize your healing hands?

Prayer:

Heavenly Father, I come before you as a vessel of healing in the lives of those I serve. May my hands be anointed with your grace and guided by your strength. Uphold me with your righteous right hand, Lord, as I embark on this journey of restoration. Help me to be a conduit of your love and compassion, bringing comfort to those in need. In Jesus' name, I pray. Amen.

Day 2: Strength in Compassionate Care

Verse of the Day:

Colossians 3:12 - "Therefore, as God's chosen people, holy and dearly loved, clothe yourselves with compassion, kindness, humility, gentleness, and patience."

Reflection:

In the field of physiotherapy, your compassionate care is a garment woven with threads of kindness and humility.

Colossians 3:12 invites you to clothe yourself in these virtues, recognizing that you are chosen, holy, and dearly loved by God. As you embark on each session, let compassion be the guiding principle that shapes your interactions and interventions.

In the tapestry of your care, weave the threads of humility, gentleness, and patience. Embrace your role as a chosen instrument of healing, reflecting God's love in every gesture.

Each act of compassion becomes an expression of God's love, echoing the virtues outlined in Colossians. As you attend to the physical needs of your patients, remember that your compassionate care has the power to uplift not only their bodies but also their spirits.

Journal:

1. How does the concept of being chosen, holy, and dearly loved by God influence your approach to providing compassionate care in your practice?

2. Reflect on a specific instance where you found strength in practicing kindness and humility during a challenging patient interaction.

3. In what ways can you intentionally cultivate a spirit of patience and gentleness in your daily interactions with patients, aligning with the virtues mentioned in Colossians 3:12?

Prayer:

Heavenly Father, as I extend compassionate care to those in need, clothe me with virtues of kindness, humility, gentleness, and patience. Let my actions be a reflection of your love and a source of comfort to those under my care. May I embrace the calling to be chosen, holy, and dearly loved, sharing these blessings with those I serve. In Jesus' name, I pray. Amen.

Day 3: Guidance in Therapeutic Strategies

Verse of the Day:

Proverbs 3:5-6 - "Trust in the LORD with all your heart and lean not on your own understanding; in all your ways submit to him, and he will make your paths straight."

Reflection:

In the intricate realm of therapeutic strategies, Proverbs 3:5-6 serves as a guiding light, encouraging you to trust in the Lord with unwavering faith.

As you embark on the journey of devising therapeutic plans, this scripture reminds you to lean not solely on your understanding but to submit each approach to the divine wisdom that makes paths straight.

As a physiotherapist, your dedication to healing aligns with the trust placed in the Lord.

Each therapeutic strategy becomes a collaborative effort between your expertise and the divine guidance that Proverbs emphasizes.

Submitting your plans to God ensures that your paths in the world of therapeutic care are directed by wisdom beyond human comprehension.

Journal:

1. How does trusting in the Lord impact your approach to devising therapeutic strategies for your patients?

2. Reflect on a specific instance where you felt divine guidance in your therapeutic decisions. What lessons did you learn from that experience?

3. In what ways can you actively submit your therapeutic plans to God, seeking alignment with His wisdom?

Prayer:

Heavenly Father, as I navigate the complexities of therapeutic strategies, I choose to trust in You with all my heart. Guide my understanding, and may Your wisdom illuminate the paths I tread in the realm of physiotherapy. I submit my plans to You, seeking Your direction and insight in every healing endeavor. In Jesus' name, I pray. Amen.

Day 4: Restoration and Renewal

Verse of the Day:

Psalm 23:3 - "He restores my soul. He leads me in paths of righteousness for his name's sake."

Reflection:

In the pursuit of healing and restoration, Psalm 23:3 offers solace and inspiration. As a physiotherapist, your mission aligns with the divine promise of soul restoration.

God leads you in paths of righteousness, guiding the therapeutic journey toward renewal for His name's sake.

In the realm of physiotherapy, where restoration is a core objective, this scripture serves as a reminder that your efforts contribute to a higher purpose. The restoration of your patients' well-being reflects God's desire for wholeness.

Embrace this divine partnership, allowing God to lead you in righteous paths as you facilitate healing and renewal in the lives you touch.

Journal:

1. How does the concept of God restoring your soul resonate with your role in physiotherapy?

2. Reflect on a moment where you witnessed significant restoration or renewal in a patient's life. How did it impact your perspective on your work?

3. In what ways can you align your therapeutic practices with God's paths of righteousness for the greater purpose of restoration?

Prayer:

Lord, I acknowledge Your role in restoring souls and leading in paths of righteousness. As I engage in the work of physiotherapy, may Your presence guide every step, bringing renewal and healing to those I serve. Use me as an instrument of Your restoration, for Your name's sake. In Jesus' name, I pray. Amen.

Day 5: Balancing Patience and Progress

Verse of the Day:

Ecclesiastes 7:8 - "The end of a matter is better than its beginning, and patience is better than pride."

Reflection:

In the intricate dance of physiotherapy, where progress is sought and healing unfolds gradually, Ecclesiastes 7:8 brings forth a timeless truth.

The journey toward the end of a matter, marked by healing and improvement, surpasses the initial stages. Patience, a virtue echoed in this scripture, stands as a beacon for your path as a physiotherapist.

As you navigate the complexities of patient care, remember that each step forward is a triumph, and the culmination of the therapeutic journey is a testament to both your dedication and the importance of patience.

Embrace the wisdom of Ecclesiastes, recognizing that true progress is often a result of patience over pride.

Journal:

1. How do you balance the desire for progress with the patience required in your role as a physiotherapist?

2. Reflect on a specific case where patience played a crucial role in achieving positive outcomes. What lessons did you learn from that experience?

3. In what ways can you cultivate a spirit of patience in your daily practice to enhance the overall progress of your patients?

Prayer:

Dear Lord, grant me the patience needed in my role as a physiotherapist. May I find joy in the journey of progress, understanding that patience is a powerful virtue in the realm of healing. Guide me to balance ambition with the wisdom to wait for the right time. Amen.

Day 6: Holistic Healing: Mind, Body, and Spirit

Verse of the Day:

1 Thessalonians 5:23 - "May God himself, the God of peace, sanctify you through and through. May your whole spirit, soul, and body be kept blameless at the coming of our Lord Jesus Christ."

Reflection:

In the pursuit of healing, 1 Thessalonians 5:23 encapsulates the essence of holistic care – an approach that encompasses the interconnectedness of the mind, body, and spirit.

As a physiotherapist, you play a vital role in facilitating this holistic healing journey. This scripture invites reflection on the profound impact that your care can have on the complete well-being of individuals.

As you attend to physical ailments, may you also consider the emotional and spiritual dimensions of health.

Embracing the holistic nature of healing can contribute not only to physical recovery but also to the peace that transcends understanding.

Journal:

1. How do you currently incorporate holistic approaches in your physiotherapy practice?

2. Reflect on a moment when addressing the spiritual or emotional aspect of a patient's well-being significantly contributed to their overall healing.

3. In what ways can you further integrate holistic care into your professional approach?

Prayer:

Lord, guide me to approach physiotherapy with a holistic mindset. May my care extend beyond the physical, embracing the interconnectedness of the mind, body, and spirit. Grant me wisdom to contribute to comprehensive healing. Amen.

Day 7: The Joy of Restoring Mobility

Verse of the Day:

Psalm 30:2 - "O LORD my God, I cried to you for help, and you have healed me."

Reflection:

In the realm of physiotherapy, Psalm 30:2 resonates with the profound joy embedded in the restoration of mobility.

Your efforts, guided by compassion and expertise, become instrumental in answering the cry for help and facilitating the healing process.

This scripture serves as a reminder that the work you do goes beyond the physical exercises; it touches the lives of individuals seeking restoration.

The joy experienced when witnessing improved mobility is a testament to the impact of your skills on the overall well-being of those in your care.

Journal:

1. Reflect on a specific moment when you witnessed the joy of a patient upon achieving improved mobility.

2. How does Psalm 30:2 influence your perspective on the significance of mobility in the healing journey?

3. In what ways can you continue fostering a positive and encouraging environment for patients during their mobility restoration?

Prayer:

Heavenly Father, thank you for the joy that comes from witnessing the restoration of mobility. Grant me continued compassion and skill to be a channel of healing for those in need. Amen.

Day 8: The Therapist's Rest: Trusting in God's Provision

Verse of the Day:

Philippians 4:19 - "And my God will supply every need of yours according to his riches in glory in Christ Jesus."

Reflection:

As a physiotherapist, you often find yourself pouring energy and care into meeting the needs of others.

Philippians 4:19 offers a comforting assurance that, just as you attend to the needs of your patients, God, in His abundance, will supply all your needs.

In the demanding and sometimes draining field of physiotherapy, this scripture invites you to lean on God's promise of provision.

Your commitment to the well-being of others aligns with the divine assurance that God, the ultimate Provider, understands your needs and stands ready to supply them.

Journal:

1. Reflect on a time when you felt physically or emotionally drained in your role. How did God provide for you during that time?

2. How does Philippians 4:19 impact your approach to work, knowing that God promises to supply your needs?

3. In what ways can you incorporate moments of rest and trust in God's provision into your daily routine?

Prayer:

I acknowledge my reliance on You for strength and sustenance in my role as a physiotherapist. Help me find rest in Your promises and trust in Your abundant provision. Amen.

Day 9: Empathy in the Healing Journey

Verse of the day:

Romans 12:15 - "Rejoice with those who rejoice; mourn with those who mourn."

Reflection:

In the realm of physiotherapy, your journey with patients encompasses both triumphs and challenges.

Romans 12:15 encourages an empathetic approach, urging you to share in the joys and sorrows of those under your care.

This scripture serves as a poignant reminder that, beyond the physical aspects of healing, your ability to connect emotionally with patients adds a profound dimension to their therapeutic journey.

Rejoicing in their progress and empathizing with their struggles reflects the compassionate care modeled by Jesus.

Journal:

1. Recall a moment when you celebrated a significant breakthrough with a patient. How did it impact your connection with them?

2. How can you incorporate a more empathetic approach in your daily interactions with patients?

3. Reflect on a challenging situation with a patient. How did you demonstrate empathy, and what could you do differently in the future?

Prayer:

Heavenly Father, grant me the ability to rejoice in moments of healing and to extend genuine empathy during times of struggle. May my actions reflect Your loving and empathetic nature. Amen.

Day 10: Walking in the Light: Honoring God Through Your Practice

Verse of the Day:

1 John 1:7 - "But if we walk in the light, as he is in the light, we have fellowship with one another, and the blood of Jesus, his Son, purifies us from all sin."

Reflection:

In the field of physiotherapy, the principles of 1 John 1:7 guide you to walk in the light, fostering fellowship and acknowledging the transformative power of Christ's sacrifice.

As a physiotherapist, your commitment to ethical and compassionate practices becomes a reflection of the light, purifying the therapeutic journey for both you and your patients.

This scripture encourages you to cultivate an environment of openness, transparency, and mutual respect.

By aligning your professional conduct with the light of God, you contribute to a healing atmosphere that goes beyond physical restoration, promoting spiritual and emotional well-being.

Journal:

1. How can you incorporate the principles of walking in the light into your daily interactions with patients and colleagues?

2. Reflect on a moment when transparency and fellowship enhanced the therapeutic process. How did it impact the outcome?

3. In what ways can your professional practice become a source of light for those you serve?

Prayer:

Gracious Lord, guide me to walk in the light of Your truth and love in my physiotherapy practice. May my actions reflect Your purity and contribute to a healing environment for both me and those under my care. Amen.

Day 11: Wisdom in Therapeutic Decision-Making

Verse of the Day:

James 1:5 - "If any of you lacks wisdom, you should ask God, who gives generously to all without finding fault, and it will be given to you."

Reflection:

In the intricate world of physiotherapy, the divine wisdom offered in James 1:5 becomes a guiding light in therapeutic decision-making. This scripture invites you to seek God's wisdom generously, trusting that it will be granted abundantly and without judgment.

As a physiotherapist, incorporating this wisdom into your practice leads to well-informed decisions that positively impact the healing journey of those under your care. Embrace the humility of seeking divine wisdom, recognizing that it surpasses human understanding.

Approach each therapeutic decision with a heart open to God's guidance, understanding that the wisdom you receive extends beyond your professional expertise.

Journal:

1. How can you intentionally seek divine wisdom in your daily therapeutic decision-making?

2. Reflect on a challenging decision you faced recently. In what ways could seeking God's wisdom have influenced the outcome?

3. How can incorporating divine wisdom enhance the effectiveness and compassion in your physiotherapy practice?

Prayer:

Heavenly Father, grant me the wisdom to make sound therapeutic decisions that align with Your divine guidance. May Your wisdom guide my hands and heart as I contribute to the healing and well-being of those entrusted to my care. Amen.

Day 12: Finding Strength in Adversity: A Therapist's Perspective

Verse of the Day:

2 Corinthians 12:9 - "But he said to me, 'My grace is sufficient for you, for my power is made perfect in weakness.'"

Reflection:

In the realm of physiotherapy, where the challenges of adversity are encountered, the scripture from 2 Corinthians 12:9 offers profound comfort.

It reminds you that in moments of weakness or difficulty, God's grace is more than sufficient. As you navigate through professional challenges, acknowledge that your strength is not solely based on personal capabilities but is perfected through reliance on divine grace.

Embrace the perspective that, in moments of adversity, God's power is uniquely revealed. Your role as a physiotherapist becomes a testament to the transformative strength found in surrendering to His grace.

This scripture invites you to draw strength from moments of weakness, recognizing that God's power operates in and through your challenges.

Journal:

1. Reflect on a challenging case or situation in your physiotherapy practice. How might embracing God's grace bring strength to your approach?

2. In what ways can acknowledging your weaknesses lead to a deeper reliance on God's power in your professional journey?

3. How can you share the lessons of finding strength in adversity with your colleagues or fellow physiotherapists?

Prayer:

Heavenly Father, in moments of adversity, I find solace in the assurance that Your grace is more than sufficient. May Your power be perfected in my weaknesses as I navigate the challenges of my physiotherapy practice. Strengthen me, and let Your grace shine through every aspect of my professional journey. Amen

Day 13: Building Trusting Therapeutic Relationships

Verse of the Day:

Proverbs 22:1 - "A good name is more desirable than great riches; to be esteemed is better than silver or gold."

Reflection:

As a physiotherapist, the foundation of your practice is built on the relationships you form with your patients.

Proverbs 22:1 emphasizes the value of a good reputation, reminding you that trust and esteem are treasures more precious than material wealth.

Each therapeutic encounter is an opportunity to nurture trust, leaving a lasting impact on the lives you touch. Consider this scripture as a guiding principle in establishing and maintaining relationships with your patients.

The pursuit of a good name is not only an ethical practice but also a reflection of the commitment to providing holistic and compassionate care. The esteem gained through trust will endure, enriching both your professional journey and the lives of those under your care.

Journal

1. How do you prioritize building trust with your patients in your daily practice?

2. Reflect on a moment when your professional reputation positively influenced a patient's experience. How did it impact their therapeutic journey?

3. In what ways can you further enhance your therapeutic relationships to reflect the value of a good name mentioned in Proverbs 22:1?

Prayer:

Heavenly Father, guide me in establishing trusting relationships with those under my care. May my actions and words reflect the value of a good name, and may Your wisdom inspire every interaction. Let the therapeutic journey be not just physical but also deeply rooted in trust and compassion. Amen.

Day 14: The Impact of Gentle Touch

Verse of the Day:

Luke 8:43-48 - "Someone touched me; I know that power has gone out from me."

Reflection:

In the realm of physiotherapy, the power of gentle touch is profound. Luke 8:43-48 recounts the healing touch of Jesus, illustrating the transformative impact of physical contact.

As a physiotherapist, you too possess the ability to bring comfort and healing through touch. This scripture serves as a reminder of the potential positive influence your hands can have on the well-being of your patients.

Reflect on the significance of touch in your therapeutic practice. In moments of gentle connection, you emulate the compassion and healing found in the scriptures.

Acknowledge the power that flows through your touch, and let it be a source of comfort and restoration for those you serve.

Journal:

1. How do you perceive the role of touch in your practice, especially in light of Luke 8:43-48?

2. Share an experience where a gentle touch positively influenced a patient's healing journey.

3. In what ways can you intentionally incorporate a compassionate touch to enhance the therapeutic experience for your patients?

Prayer:

Heavenly Father, grant me the wisdom to recognize the healing potential in the gift of touch. May my hands be instruments of comfort and restoration, reflecting Your compassionate touch in every therapeutic encounter. Amen.

Day 15: Serving with Compassionate Listening

Verse of the Day:

James 1:19 - "My dear brothers and sisters, take note of this: Everyone should be quick to listen, slow to speak, and slow to become angry."

Reflection:

In the symphony of healing, the art of compassionate listening is a powerful instrument. James 1:19 encourages us to be attentive listeners, quick to understand, slow to respond, and patient in our interactions.

As a physiotherapist, your ability to listen empathetically can profoundly impact the therapeutic journey of your patients. Consider the significance of listening in your practice.

Cultivate an environment where your patients feel heard and understood, just as our Creator listens to our hearts. Recognize that through attentive listening, you not only address physical ailments but also provide emotional and spiritual support.

Journal:

1. Reflect on a moment when your attentive listening positively influenced a patient's experience.

2. How can you enhance your listening skills to create a more compassionate therapeutic environment?

3. In what ways can you integrate the principles of James 1:19 into your daily practice?

Prayer:

Heavenly Father, grant me the ability to listen with a compassionate heart. May my ears be attuned to the needs of my patients, offering not only physical healing but also emotional and spiritual support. Help me embody the virtues of patience and understanding in my practice. Amen.

Day 16: Promoting Wellness in All Aspects of Life

Verse of the Day:

3 John 1:2 - "Dear friend, I pray that you may enjoy good health and that all may go well with you, even as your soul is getting along."

Reflection:

In the pursuit of holistic healing, 3 John 1:2 serves as a reminder to address well-being in its entirety. As a physiotherapist, your role extends beyond the physical to promote wellness in every aspect of life.

Consider the interconnectedness of physical health, mental well-being, and the flourishing of the soul in your practice. Acknowledge the impact of your therapeutic interventions on the overall wellness of your patients.

Embrace the prayerful sentiment of 3 John 1:2, not only for your patients but also for yourself. Strive to contribute to the improvement of their physical health while fostering a sense of harmony and well-being that extends to the soul.

Journal:

1. How do you currently integrate wellness practices into your physiotherapy approach?

2. Reflect on a moment when you witnessed a positive transformation in a patient's overall well-being.

3. In what ways can you further promote holistic wellness in your practice, aligning with the principles of 3 John 1:2?

Prayer:

Gracious God, guide me in promoting wellness in the lives of those under my care. May my efforts contribute not only to physical healing but also to the flourishing of the soul. Grant me wisdom to embrace a holistic approach, recognizing the interconnected aspects of health. Amen.

Day 17: Finding Joy in the Healing Process

Verse of the Day:

Psalm 126:5 - "Those who sow with tears will reap with songs of joy."

Reflection:

As a physiotherapist, the healing journey often involves perseverance through challenging moments.

Psalm 126:5 reminds us that even in times of tears and struggle, there is a promise of joy in the reaping. Consider the joy that emerges in the healing process, both for your patients and yourself, as progress is made and hurdles are overcome.

Embrace the transformative power of joy within the healing journey. Reflect on the moments of triumph and progress, recognizing that they are seeds sown in tears that blossom into songs of joy.

Let this scripture guide your perspective, infusing your practice with an understanding that the challenges are an integral part of the eventual joyous outcome.

Journal:

1. How do you currently celebrate small victories and moments of progress in your practice?

2. Reflect on a specific case where you witnessed the joy of healing emerging from challenging circumstances.

3. In what ways can you intentionally bring joy into the therapeutic process, aligning with the spirit of Psalm 126:5?

Prayer:

Heavenly Father, grant me the ability to find joy in the healing journey, both for my patients and myself. May the tears sown in challenging moments lead to a harvest of songs of joy. Guide me in fostering an environment where healing is accompanied by a spirit of celebration. Amen.

Day 18: Holiness in Healthcare: A Therapist's Mission

Verse of the Day:

Colossians 3:17 - "And whatever you do, whether in word or deed, do it all in the name of the Lord Jesus, giving thanks to God the Father through him.

Reflection:

In the sacred realm of healthcare, Colossians 3:17 serves as a guiding light for physiotherapists. Your work, whether in words or actions, becomes a mission undertaken in the name of the Lord Jesus.

Embrace the profound responsibility to bring healing and wholeness to others, recognizing that each therapeutic interaction is an opportunity to express gratitude to God.

Infuse your practice with holiness, understanding that the work you do is a reflection of your faith. As a physiotherapist, you are called to honor the Lord in every aspect of your service.

Consider how the principles of Colossians 3:17 can deepen your sense of purpose, transforming your daily work into a mission that goes beyond physical rehabilitation.

Journal:

1. How can you incorporate the principles of Colossians 3:17 into your daily interactions with patients?

2. Reflect on a specific moment where you felt the presence of God in your therapeutic work.

3. In what ways can you consciously give thanks to God through your professional practice?

Prayer:

Heavenly Father, guide me in living out Colossians 3:17 in my role as a physiotherapist. May every word spoken and every action taken in my practice be a reflection of Your name. Thank You for the opportunity to bring healing and wholeness to others. Amen.

Day 19: Adapting to Change in Healthcare

Verse of the Day:

Isaiah 43:19 - "See, I am doing a new thing! Now it springs up; do you not perceive it? I am making a way in the wilderness and streams in the wasteland."

Reflection:

In the ever-evolving landscape of healthcare, Isaiah 43:19 serves as a source of encouragement for physiotherapists.

Embrace the inevitability of change, recognizing that the Lord is constantly at work, bringing forth new opportunities and possibilities. As you navigate the challenges of the healthcare environment, trust that God is making a way, even in seemingly barren circumstances.

Reflect on how this scripture can inspire you to perceive and welcome the new things unfolding in your professional journey.

Consider the transformative impact that adaptation can have on your practice, allowing streams of innovation and resilience to flow through the often challenging healthcare wilderness.

Journal:

1. How have you experienced change in your healthcare practice, and how did you perceive God's guidance in those moments?

2. In what ways can you embrace and adapt to new opportunities and challenges in your physiotherapy work?

3. Consider a time when you witnessed positive transformation in your healthcare environment. How did it impact your perspective on change?

Prayer:

Heavenly Father, grant me the wisdom and discernment to perceive the new things You are doing in my healthcare practice. Help me embrace change with faith and trust, knowing that You are making a way even in challenging circumstances. Amen.

Day 20: Grace in Therapeutic Failures

Verse of the Day:

Romans 8:28 - "And we know that in all things God works for the good of those who love him, who have been called according to his purpose."

Reflection:

In the face of therapeutic failures, Romans 8:28 offers solace and perspective for physiotherapists. Recognize that even in moments of disappointment, God is at work for the good of those who love Him.

Therapeutic setbacks can be stepping stones to growth and better outcomes, aligning with God's purpose for your journey. Reflect on how this scripture can guide you through challenges and disappointments in your therapeutic practice.

Consider the ways in which God's overarching purpose can bring meaning and redemption to moments that seem discouraging.

Journal:

1. How do you typically respond to therapeutic failures, and how might this scripture shift your perspective?

2. In what ways can you trust that God is working for the good, even in moments of professional disappointment?

3. Reflect on a specific instance where you witnessed positive outcomes emerge from a therapeutic setback.

Prayer:

Heavenly Father, in moments of therapeutic disappointment, help me trust that You are working for the good according to Your purpose. Grant me grace and resilience as I navigate challenges, knowing that Your plan is unfolding in every aspect of my practice. Amen.

Day 21: A Therapist's Legacy of Compassion

Verse of the Day:

Matthew 25:40 - "The King will reply, 'Truly I tell you, whatever you did for one of the least of these brothers and sisters of mine, you did for me.'"

Reflection:

As a physiotherapist, consider the profound impact of your compassionate care, echoing the words of Matthew 25:40.

Each act of kindness and healing is not just a professional duty but a reflection of your service to the King. Your legacy is woven into the lives you touch, embodying the essence of Christ's love.

Reflect on the scripture's message and ponder how your therapeutic interventions extend beyond physical restoration.

Contemplate the enduring legacy you're crafting through your compassionate approach to healthcare.

Journal:

1. How does the scripture influence your perspective on the significance of your therapeutic work?

2. In what ways can you consciously integrate compassion into your daily practice, aligning with the essence of Matthew 25:40?

3. Reflect on a memorable experience where you felt a profound connection between your therapeutic care and the teachings of this scripture.

Prayer:

Gracious Father, guide me in leaving a legacy of compassion through my therapeutic endeavors. May my actions reflect Your love, and may I always recognize the divine significance in each act of care. Amen.

Conclusion

As we conclude this 21-day journey, I commend you, dedicated physiotherapist, for your unwavering commitment to the well-being of others. Your journey is more than a profession; it's a sacred calling to be a conduit of healing.

In these reflections, you've not only explored the intricacies of your craft but also discovered the profound connection between your therapeutic touch and the divine source of all restoration.

May this conclusion resonate as a resounding affirmation of the impact you make daily. In the tapestry of healthcare, your compassionate efforts are threads of hope, resilience, and transformation.

Embrace the truth that your healing hands are instruments through which the divine presence manifests, bringing comfort, strength, and renewal to those in your care.

As you continue your noble work, remember that you are part of something greater – a legacy of compassion and care.

The healing journey doesn't end here; it's an ongoing expedition where you, as a physiotherapist, play a vital role.

May your steps be guided by wisdom, your touch infused with grace, and your heart filled with the knowledge that your labor of love reverberates far beyond the physical realms.

With gratitude for your service and a heart full of hope, step forward into each new day, knowing that your calling is a beacon of light in the lives you touch.

In faith and gratitude,

Delightful Devotionals